DON'T GET SUNBURNED

DON'T GET SUN BURNED

50 WAYS TO SAVE YOUR SKIN

Buck Tilton

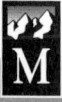
THE MOUNTAINEERS BOOKS

THE MOUNTAINEERS BOOKS
is the nonprofit publishing arm of The Mountaineers Club, an organization founded in 1906 and dedicated to the exploration, preservation, and enjoyment of outdoor and wilderness areas.

1001 SW Klickitat Way, Suite 201, Seattle, WA 98134

© 2009 by Buck Tilton

All rights reserved

First edition, 2009

No part of this book may be reproduced in any form, or by any electronic, mechanical, or other means, without permission in writing from the publisher.

Manufactured in the United States of America

Copy Editor: Joeth Zucco
Cover and Layout: Peggy Egerdahl
Illustrator: Marge Mueller, Gray Mouse Graphics

Cover photograph: Colored pair of sunglasses © PeapPop, 2007. Used under license from Shutterstock.com;
Illustration: Sun © Dic Liew, 2007. Used under license from Shutterstock.com

Library of Congress Cataloging-in-Publication Data
Tilton, Buck.
 Don't get sunburned : 50 ways to save your skin / by Buck Tilton. — 1st ed.
   p. cm.
 Includes index.
 ISBN-13: 978-1-59485-105-6
 ISBN-10: 1-59485-105-0
 1. Sunburn—Popular works. I. Title.
 RL248.T55 2009
 616.5'15—dc22
                            2008047016

 Printed on recycled paper

CONTENTS

Introduction 9

Chapter 1. **UV: KNOW THE ENEMY** 19
   Be SunWise: UV Index and UV Alerts 19
   Know Solar Noon 21
   Be Aware of Sunburn Times 22
   Avoid Cloud Illusions 23
   Follow the Changing Seasons 24
   Do Not Fry High 25
   Avoid a Reflection on You 26
   Let Your Latitude Determine Your Attitude 27
   Watch the Wind 28
   Be Mindful of Midday Exposure 29
   Remember: Pollution Is Not the Solution 30
   See Through the Protection of Glass 30

Chapter 2. **UV AND SKIN DAMAGE** 32
   Know Your Skin Type 32
   Don't Get Sunburned 33
   Slow Skin Aging 35
   Beware of Basal Cell Carcinoma 36
   Search Yourself for Squamous Cell Carcinoma 37
   Monitor Yourself for Malignant Melanoma 39
   Keep an Eye on Solar Keratoses 42

    Avoid Photosensitivity Reactions   43
    Protect Your Immune System   45

Chapter 3. **UV AND SKIN PROTECTION**   47
    Do Not Trust Water to Put Out the Fire   47
    Think Twice Before Tanning   48
    Understand SPF   49
    Understand the *New* UVA Rating System   50
    Use Sunscreen   51
    Apply Sunscreens Correctly   53
    Block the Sun   54
    Don't Give the Sun Any Lip   55
    Dress for the Sun: Part 1   56
    Dress for the Sun: Part 2   57
    Wear the Right Hat   58

Chapter 4. **UV AND EYE PROTECTION**   60
    Wear Sunglasses: Prevent Solar Retinitis   60
    Wear Sunglasses: Prevent Cataracts   61
    Wear Sunglasses: Prevent Snow Blindness   62
    Wear Sunglasses!   63
    Understand Labels on Sunglasses   65
    Test Your Sunglasses   66
    Consider Prescription Sunglasses   67
    Consider Overglasses   68

Chapter 5. UV: MORE GOOD THINGS TO DO 70
- Be Vacation-Wise 70
- Do Not Mix Babies and Bright Sunlight 71
- Teach Your Children Well 73
- Use a UV Meter 74
- Create More Shade in Your Backyard 75
- Use Portable Shade 76
- Boot the Booth 77
- Consume Enough Beta-Carotene and Vitamins C and E 78

Chapter 6. SAVE THE OZONE 80
- Do Not Buy Ozone-Eating Chemicals 80
- Help Reclaim Ozone-Depleting Chemicals 82

Appendices 84
- The Ten UV Protection Essentials 84
- Resources 84

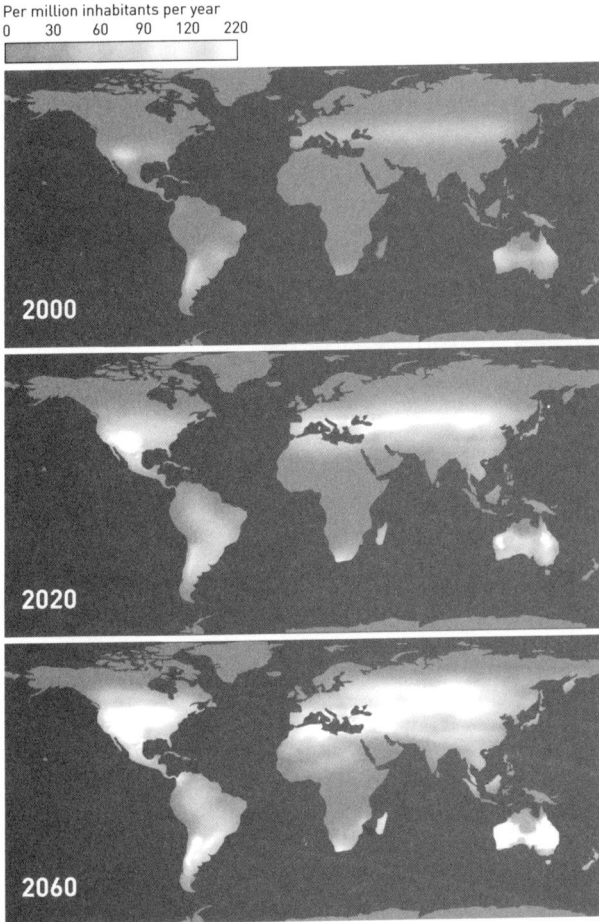

Source: Dutch National Institute for Public Health and the Environment (RIVM), Laboratory for Radiation Research, 2007.

INTRODUCTION

Sunlight is, as almost everyone knows, absolutely necessary for life as we know it to exist, but that is a topic for another book. This book is about sunlight and human skin, and about how contact between the two is not absolutely necessary for life as we know it.

Just about everybody loves the feel of the sun—on their face, on their shoulders, on their back. We are drawn to sunlight like a moth to flame. Sunlight, unlike rain, snow, sleet, hail, and wind, is certainly one reason we want to be outdoors. And yes, there are benefits, including radiant warmth, especially nice on a chilly day, and stimulation of the skin to synthesize vitamin D. Problems arise, however—and more and more often—not because we expose ourselves to sunlight but because we *overexpose* ourselves.

Solar radiation—a fancy word for sunlight—reaches Earth in rays of many different wavelengths. Some we can see with our eyes (visible light), and some are invisible (infrared and ultraviolet light). Some we can feel on our skin as heat (infrared), and some we cannot feel at all (visible and ultraviolet). Wavelengths are measured

---

Opposite: *Skin cancer, the most common cancer on Earth, is also the fastest growing type of cancer, with more than one million new cases reported each year in the United States alone.*

in nanometers (nm). The chart below compares the wavelengths of sunlight:

Above 700 nm	Infrared (invisible)
650–700 nm	Red light (visible)
590–650 nm	Orange light (visible)
490–590 nm	Yellow and Green light (visible)
420–490 nm	Blue light (visible)
400–420 nm	Violet light (visible)
320–400 nm	Ultraviolet A (invisible)
280–320 nm	Ultraviolet B (invisible)
Below 280 nm	Ultraviolet C (invisible)

ABOUT UV LIGHT AND OZONE

Ultraviolet (UV) rays, the shorter wavelengths, the waves we are concerned about in this book, can actually damage living cells. The shortest of the shorter UV wavelengths are the most damaging, containing enough energy to destroy DNA molecules in your skin and eyes. DNA is the genetic stuff that genes are made of, and genes control cell health and growth. If the genetic material is damaged severely enough, cells begin to grow in the disorderly manner known as cancer. UV radiation, in other words, is the main cause of skin cancer.

Global warming, fact or fiction, has captured the attention of most of us, causing at least some people to forget that skin cancer rates continue to rise dramatically. The rise in cancer sufferers is primarily due to an increase in outdoor recreational lifestyles, but experts remain concerned about another cause of increased ultraviolet radiation exposure: the thinning of Earth's natural, protective ozone shield, allowing more and more UV light through. (And there may well be a relationship between ozone depletion and global warming.) To help you better understand the increase in health hazards related to UV light and ozone depletion, let's review some history and science.

Ozone, a blue gas with a pungent odor, takes its name from the Greek word *ozon* meaning "smell." This gas was discovered in the 1840s by Christian Friedrich Schönbein at the University of Basel, Switzerland. Most of our ozone, about 90 percent, lies in the stratosphere, located between 6 and 25 miles above the earth's surface. In the early 1880s scientists identified stratospheric ozone as a shield, and understood that for eons it had allowed life on Earth to flourish by passing the longer, beneficial wavelengths

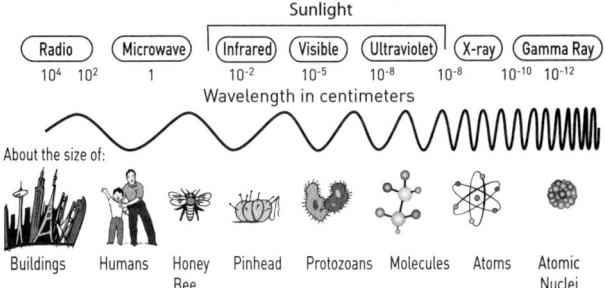

Sunlight consists of the entire electromagnetic spectrum of light, but only the shorter wavelengths harm human skin.

(heat and visible light) and effectively blocking the shorter and most dangerous UV waves.

Compared to quantities of other gases (oxygen, nitrogen, and carbon dioxide) and despite the fact that they provide a critical protective function, ozone molecules are rare in our atmosphere. The stratospheric ozone shield is a thin layer of ozone molecules—a *very* thin layer. If all the ozone molecules over our heads were compressed together with sea level pressure, they would form a layer less than ⅛ inch (3 millimeters) thick, about the thickness of the filling in a Fig Newton. Mighty thin, yes, but ozone has unique optical properties that permit it to serve as a shield from dangerous UV radiation.

An ozone molecule consists of three oxygen atoms. Ozone is formed in the upper atmosphere by the action of sunlight on ordinary oxygen (O_2) molecules. Sunlight splits apart some oxygen molecules into single oxygen atoms. These atoms then bond to nearby oxygen molecules creating the three-atom ozone (O_3) molecule. While this mechanism creates new ozone molecules, chemical reactions with naturally occurring compounds are constantly destroying ozone. Normally, the delicate balance in the thickness of the ozone shield has been maintained with only minor fluctuations due to sunspots or volcanic activity.

THE OZONE SHIELD: UP CLOSE AND SUFFERING

Almost all UVA radiation passes through the ozone shield, and as far as science is concerned, it always has. Ozone effectively blocks nearly all UVC. It also does a good job of

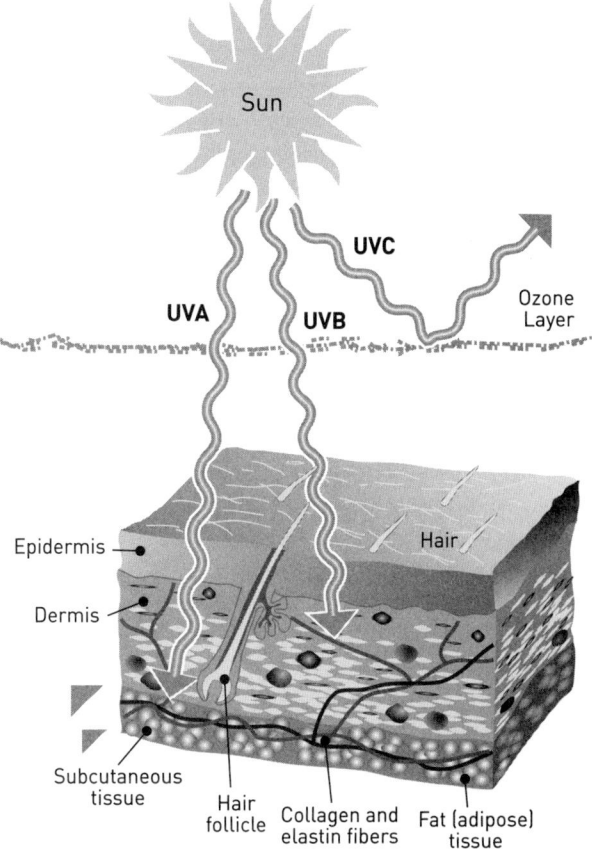

The deeper UV radiation penetrates your skin, the greater the chance of permanent damage.

protecting us from excessive UVB radiation—if the shield is undamaged and can do its job.

Ultraviolet light, being high in energy, breaks down most airborne, manmade compounds into elemental atoms at low altitudes above the earth's surface. Manmade chemicals, therefore, have been rare or absent in the stratosphere—until the invention of halocarbons. Halocarbons are so stable they do not break down before they reach the stratosphere. All halocarbons contain either chlorine or bromine and included among them are halons, carbon tetrachloride, and methyl chloroform. But the best-known halocarbons are chlorofluorocarbons (CFCs), used for years in refrigeration, air conditioning, plastic foams, and as industrial cleaners. CFCs were invented by the DuPont Corporation in the 1930s and sold under the trademarked name Freon. Nontoxic and noncombustible, CFCs, at that time, appeared to be "ideal chemicals."

Then, in 1974, Sherry Rowland and Mario Molina, chemists working at the University of California at Irvine, announced that CFCs could be a potential threat to the ozone layer. They showed that if CFCs released their chlorine atoms in the stratosphere, this extra chlorine could become a catalyst to greatly accelerate ozone destruction. These two chemists produced in their laboratory the ozone-destroying reactions they feared were occurring in the upper atmosphere, but their warnings were ignored by the chemical industry and the government. CFC production continued to increase.

It was a team of British scientists, and not until 1985, who first measured an undeniable and significant drop in the level of stratospheric ozone (at their Antarctic research station at Halley Bay). The reductions were *very* dramatic during the month of October, springtime in Antarctica. Soon NASA's Nimbus series of satellites confirmed the ozone loss, and full-color images were generated of what became known as the Antarctic Ozone Hole. (An ozone hole, by the way, is not a true hole with no ozone but an area of extreme ozone depletion.) Now scientists needed to determine if the ozone loss was due to CFCs as Roland and Molina suspected. In August and September of 1987, NASA used high-altitude aircraft to fly through the hole while measuring the levels of chlorine and ozone. The results left no doubt: CFCs were at least the primary cause of ozone depletion.

Since that discovery, governments around the world have joined in an unprecedented global effort to first slow and then stop the production of CFCs (and halons). The Montreal Protocol in 1988 was the first step, calling for reduced CFC production. But during the years immediately following the 1985 discovery, ozone levels worldwide continued to drop, and the Protocol was revised with the London (1990) and then the Copenhagen (1992) Amendments. Under the Copenhagen Amendment, most CFC production was phased out by 1996, but other dangerous chlorine compounds will not be phased out until the year 2015, and some chemicals with the potential to destroy ozone are still not regulated at all.

In 2001 NASA confirmed an ozone hole was opening on the opposite side of our planet, and in 2005 established without a doubt that it was growing. Scientists suspect the Arctic Ozone Hole will continue to grow until at least 2020.

In 2006 the size of the Antarctic Ozone Hole reached its largest ever, covering an area more than three times the size of the United States. In 2007 the size of the hole shrank by approximately 30 percent.

Ozone holes, as you can see, are not static—they grow and shrink seasonally and annually and change due to the temperature of the atmosphere and the amount of solar radiation striking the earth—but they are anticipated to periodically cover larger and larger areas in the next few years.

THE FUTURE

Since the discovery of the Antarctic Ozone Hole and the birth of worldwide concern over ozone depletion, scientists have labored to discover, but still do not fully understand, what will happen to our ozone shield in the future. However, a few basic facts are known: Ozone-destroying chemicals are still rising into the stratosphere, and they will continue to rise for a few more years, even if we stop production of all dangerous chemicals immediately (which we have *not* done). Ozone levels, overall, are decreasing on a worldwide basis, currently at a rate of about 4 percent per year. As ozone levels decrease, measured UVB levels are on the rise, and can be expected to keep on rising in years to come. And increases in UV levels

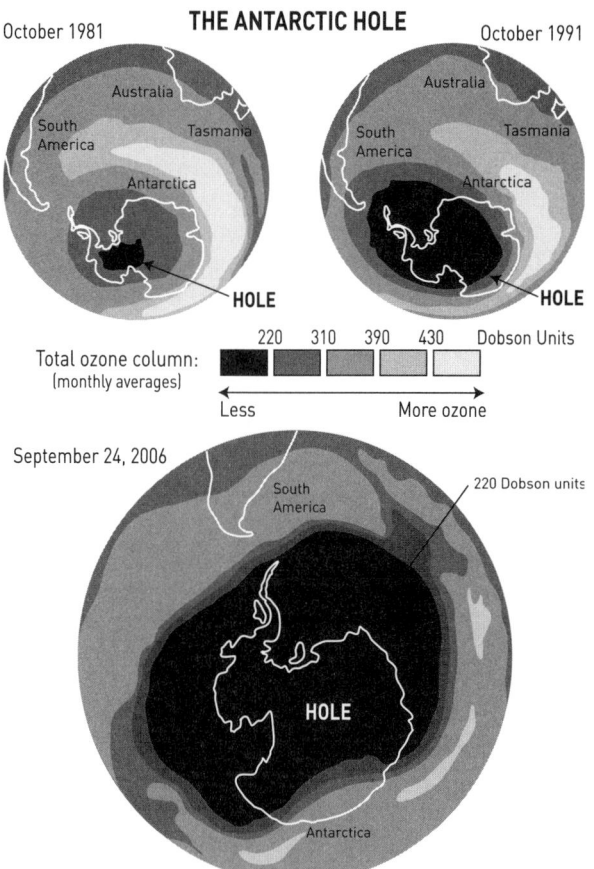

Holes, where ozone has dropped alarmingly in volume, vary in size from year to year, but the Antarctic Hole has grown overall in staggering leaps since 1981. From September 21 to 30, 2006, its average area was the largest ever observed.

Source: U.S. National Oceanic and Atmospheric Administration (NOAA), 2007.

cause an increase in the threat to human skin.

With the increased threat—and since ozone levels fluctuate in seasonal patterns, depending on latitude, and drop rapidly during ozone hole episodes—some governments, including ours, have begun to include UV radiation forecasts as a standard part of daily local weather forecasts. How to use those forecasts is explained in this book—as are forty-nine other ways to save your skin.

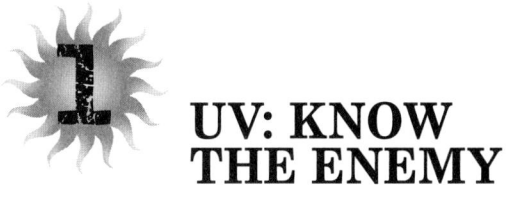

UV: KNOW THE ENEMY

IMAGINE THIS:
Summer vacation in the mountains of Colorado, and the July midday temps are comfortably lower than back home. Even better, a cooling breeze moves beneath a mass of clouds that shade the ground. You're not worried about sunburn—are you?

BE SUNWISE: UV INDEX AND UV ALERTS
Here is a fact you should know: There is a UV Index. Developed by the National Weather Service (NWS) and the U.S. Environmental Protection Agency (EPA), the UV Index predicts the intensity level of ultraviolet radiation and provides a forecast of the risk you face from overexposure to the sun. The UV Index gives you a number on a scale from 1 to 11+, with 1 indicating a low risk of overexposure and 11+ an extreme risk. The number represents the maximum level of UV radiation for the day, which occurs at solar noon (see Know Solar Noon). The number is painstakingly generated for the next four days for every zip code of the United States from data collected by satellites and run through a computer model. The UV Index takes into account local conditions (ozone levels, cloud formations, and elevation

above sea level) that affect the amount of UV radiation reaching the ground. The UV Index is available at www.epa.gov/sunwise/uvindex.html.

UV Index	Exposure Level	Message
1–2	Low	Safely enjoy sunlight. Wear sunglasses on bright days. If you burn easily, cover up and use sunscreen of SPF 15 or more.
3–5	Moderate	Precautions are recommended. Wear a hat and use sunscreen, reduce exposure during midday.
6–8	High	Precautions are needed. Wear a wide-brimmed hat and sunglasses, and long-sleeved shirt and pants when practical. Use sunscreen of SPF 15 or higher. Avoid the midday sun.
8–10	Very High	Avoid direct sunlight whenever possible, especially between 10 AM and 4 PM. A shirt, a hat, and sunscreen are musts.
11+	Extreme	Maximum protection against the sun is demanded. Seek shade whenever possible.

The SunWise website, a service of the EPA, provides valuable tips on protecting your skin as well as whether or not a UV Alert is in effect. The EPA issues a UV Alert when the UV radiation predicted to strike your area will be 6 or higher on the UV Index and when this level of intensity is unusual for the time of year.

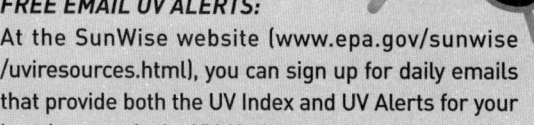

FREE EMAIL UV ALERTS:
At the SunWise website (www.epa.gov/sunwise/uviresources.html), you can sign up for daily emails that provide both the UV Index and UV Alerts for your location or only the UV Alerts.

What To Do
Understand the UV Index and take preventive measures to match the risk. Watch for a UV Alert and heed its warning: Take *extra* care to protect your skin.

KNOW SOLAR NOON
The sun's rays strike the earth at maximum intensity when the sun stands at its highest point in the sky (the nearest zenith) above you. This occurs at midday, exactly halfway between sunrise and sunset, a time known as "solar noon," when the damaging effects of UV radiation reach their most dangerous. Solar noon usually does *not* occur at exactly 12 PM local time. It varies with your location, the time of year, and whether or not your location is on Standard Time or Daylight Savings Time. For example, solar noon occurred in Atlanta, Georgia, on January 16, 2008, at 12:47:01 PM.

What To Do

The exact time of solar noon is available on the solar calculator of the National Oceanic and Atmospheric Administration (NOAA) at www.srrb.noaa.gov. You can estimate solar noon fairly accurately by calculating the length of the upcoming daylight from sunrise and sunset (check your local newspaper) and dividing by two. It is best to remain indoors or in the deepest shade available during the period surrounding solar noon.

BE AWARE OF SUNBURN TIMES

Here is the question: How long does it take for skin to sunburn? The answer, unfortunately, depends on numerous variables including skin type, ozone level, cloud cover, and elevation above sea level (and these factors are all discussed in this book). When you know the UV Index for your location, you can guess—from the chart below—the amount of exposure time it will take to sunburn your skin. The sunburn times in the chart are an estimate of how many minutes pass before the first noticeable reddening occurs on Type III skin, which the American Melanoma Foundation refers to as "average skin" (see Know Your Skin Type). Remember that more sensitive skin types will burn in a shorter time while people with darker skin can tolerate longer exposures. (For more on sunburn, see Don't Get Sunburned).

UV Index	Sunburn Times
1–3	60+ minutes
4–6	40–60 minutes
7–9	30–40 minutes
10+	less than 30 minutes

What To Do

Since sunburn times vary, sometimes altering quickly with changing conditions, the safest bet is to take precautions against sunburn whenever your skin will be exposed.

AVOID CLOUD ILLUSIONS

Most clouds, for all their wondrous variety and despite the fact they provide some shade, share a common failing: They absorb less UV radiation than you probably think. You are probably well aware that a cloudy day may be no protection from sunburn. Depending on the individual cloud, the amount of UV radiation absorbed can range from almost none to around 80 percent, but only rarely will the amount absorbed reach 40 percent. Thick, dark rain clouds offer significant protection, protection you are likely to *not* need since you may be covered with rainwear. Clouds *do* block heat-packing infrared rays, however, and so they cool the air. Since you feel cooler, you are typically not as aware of the burning effect of UV radiation. On a bright day with fluffy cumulus clouds overhead, you can actually receive an increased dose of UVB—sometimes up to and occasionally beyond 15 percent more—because these white clouds reflect scattered UV radiation down to earth.

What To Do
Do not ever rely on clouds to protect your skin—or your eyes. Wear a brimmed hat, sunscreen, and sunglasses under cloudy skies—unless, of course, you are already in a raincoat and/or under an umbrella.

FOLLOW THE CHANGING SEASONS
UV radiation levels depend on both the seasonal strength of the sun and the seasonal thickness of the ozone shield. Although the sun stands closer to the earth in winter, it is more directly overhead in summer. Summertime in North America brings more sunshine, warmer weather, and the highest levels of UV radiation of the year.

The longest day of the year occurs at the summer solstice—usually June 21—but UV levels do not peak in most of the United States until sometime in mid-July. The cause of the mid-July peak is the seasonal fluctuation of ozone levels. Ozone levels are highest in early spring. They drop during the summer, reaching their lowest levels in November or December. Ozone depletion studies have revealed reductions in ozone values during all seasons, but the biggest reductions have consistently occurred in the spring months in the United States and Canada.

The range of UV fluctuation from summer to winter depends on the latitude of your location. The UV Index in San Francisco, for example, typically peaks around 8.8 in July and drops to just below 2 in December and January.

In Tampa, Florida, the UV Index hits a high of 10 in July, stays above 9 for about twelve weeks, and drops to about 4 in December.

What To Do
Be especially careful to protect your skin from the sun from early March through October.

DO NOT FRY HIGH
Here is the short version: The higher you are in elevation above sea level, the more UV radiation you receive.

Most ozone, as mentioned earlier in this book, resides in the stratosphere, but some of it can be found in our air at all altitudes. The amount of UV radiation kept from Earth's surface is determined by the *total* amount of ozone, from ground level to the upper stratosphere. Scientists call all the ozone in the air the "total ozone column." At higher elevations there is less total atmosphere above your head—and so the total ozone column reading goes lower as you go higher. Less ozone equals more UV radiation.

Experts have agreed, although not unanimously, that for every 1000 feet of elevation gained, UV radiation increases by 4–5 percent. This percentage of increase is supported by the National Weather Service. Flagstaff, Arizona, for instance, stands approximately 6000 feet higher in elevation than Phoenix, and thus receives, according to this formula, about 27 percent more UV radiation than Phoenix.

Another formula, this one the result of a more recent study, measured UVB at 500-foot intervals in the mountains of Colorado and reported an increase of 8–10 percent for every 1000 feet gained. That would make the UV radiation hitting Flagstaff in the neighborhood of 60 percent more than Phoenix. It is likely that no exact percentage of increased risk exists—but an increased risk most assuredly *does* exist.

What To Do

When out skiing, hiking, or otherwise recreating at higher elevations, remember you are receiving an increased dose of UV radiation. Wear a hat, cover your neck, and be sure your sunglasses or goggles offer side protection.

AVOID A REFLECTION ON YOU

UV radiation, being light, is reflected, as light will be, from numerous surfaces. The damaging effects of UV radiation, therefore, may be increased when the rays are reflected from anything from bright metal and white-painted surfaces to natural surfaces.

Although you have experienced the blinding reflection of sunlight from water, water actually ranks as a poor bouncer of UV radiation. At midday, with the sun directly overhead, the rays penetrate beneath the surface of water, with 5 percent or less being reflected. In early morning and toward evening, with the sun near the horizon, the amount of rays reflected increases, but by that time of day the UV radiation is low. Ice and snow, on the other hand, are good reflectors. Snow is about four times more reflective than desert sand, and clean snow can reflect up to 85 percent of UV light.

What To Do
Remember that shade may not be as protective as you think. If you are working or playing on or near reflective surfaces, protect your skin with sunscreens and clothing, and your eyes with sunglasses. Do not forget to protect the bottom of your nose and chin where reflected UV radiation can reach with surprising intensity.

LET YOUR LATITUDE DETERMINE YOUR ATTITUDE
Jimmy Buffet and your fifth grade geography teacher were both right: There is more sunlight in Mexico than in Chicago. Locations close to the equator receive the most annual sunshine, while areas close to the poles receive relatively small amounts of solar radiation. This is due to the angle of the sun varying with latitude. In polar areas the sun is always low on the horizon, while at the equator the sun is high in the sky every day, and it shines intensely.

Stronger sunlight means higher levels of UV radiation and its cancer-causing potential. The annual UVB dosage level in Dallas, as an example, is approximately 38 percent higher than in Boston. Stronger UV rays translate directly to more cases of skin cancer. There have been 47 percent more cases of skin cancer reported in Dallas than in Boston. Researchers from the U.S. Department of Health, Education, and Welfare (HEW), Public Health Service, and National Institutes of Health (NIH) tabulated the skin cancer rates for white males on a state-by-state basis. Then they plotted the cancer rates for each state according to the *latitude* for each individual state. Cancer rates in the southern states of Texas and Florida are approximately twice as high as the rates for the northern states of Wisconsin and Montana. The connection between high UVB and high cancer rates is well documented.

What To Do

As you travel south, stay aware of higher UV levels associated with these lower latitudes. It is easier to get bad sunburns in these warmer regions—even during the winter months.

WATCH THE WIND

Wind, all by itself, does not cause your skin to burn, although it can cause drying and chapping. But wind and UV radiation at the same time work together to make your sunburn worse. A term for the ill effects of wind and sun is "windburn." The combination of wind and sun can be harmful due to the following:

- the acceleration of the drying of sweat from your skin, which removes urocanic acid, a naturally occurring chemical in your skin that helps protect you from UV radiation;
- the feeling of coolness that wind produces, causing you to expose your skin to the sun longer than you otherwise would; and
- the irritative effect of wind on skin that intensifies sunburn.

What To Do

Cover up (even a light windshirt will do) when you are exposed to high wind and direct sunlight.

BE MINDFUL OF MIDDAY EXPOSURE

When is the best time to be indoors or in deep shade? Many experts say you should try to avoid direct sun exposure between the hours of 10 AM and 3 PM—and some say it is even better to avoid direct sunlight until after 4 PM. Another rule of thumb is to avoid being outdoors under direct solar radiation for the two hours before solar noon and the two hours after solar noon. At other hours of the day, the sun may be only 70 percent as strong as its highest intensity at solar noon (see Know Solar Noon). If you avoid exposure for three hours before, and three hours after solar noon, you will only be exposed to UV levels less than *half* as intense as midday levels.

What To Do

Since it is easier to get sunburned in the middle of the day, you can reduce your UV exposure risks by scheduling some of your regular outdoor activities in the morning or late afternoon. This is especially true in the late spring and during the summer months when midday UV levels are very high. For example, if your summer exercise routine includes a jog or bike ride, you could greatly reduce your UV dosage and health risks by shifting these activities from your lunch hour to before or after work.

When hiking or backpacking in the spring and summer months, take a long lunch break (or a short nap) in a shady spot to avoid the heat and high UV radiation of the midday sun.

REMEMBER: POLLUTION IS NOT THE SOLUTION

While most ozone resides in the stratospheric ozone layer miles above our heads, there is also ozone located near ground level. The low-level ozone is called tropospheric ozone. Most tropospheric ozone is created by industrial pollution and automobile exhaust gases and is called *smog*. Tropospheric ozone levels are much higher in large, congested urban areas than in rural areas.

Measurements in some large cities show the additional ozone created at ground level has partially compensated for the thinning of the stratospheric ozone layer, resulting in only small increases in UV levels. That sounds like good news—a manmade ozone shield—but, unfortunately, this is not the case. Ozone is a nasty pollutant when it occurs at ground level. Exposure to ozone causes eye irritation, lung damage, and other health problems.

What To Do

Do not rely on urban air pollution to save your skin from UV rays; you will be subjecting yourself to additional health risks in heavily polluted, high-traffic urban areas. When vacationing in rural and wilderness areas, remember to protect your skin with proper clothing and sunscreen—the sun's UV rays are stronger without the blanket of urban smog.

SEE THROUGH THE PROTECTION OF GLASS

Glass provides protection from UV radiation in varying degrees. Clear car window glass blocks about 97 percent of UVB and 37 percent of UVA. With long-term exposure, your skin could theoretically be damaged. If the glass is laminated, however, all UVB and about 80 percent of UVA is blocked. Behind a windshield coated with clear film, 97 percent of UVA is blocked. Overall, then, you are safe in a car, unless your arm hangs out an open window for hours—or you have the top down on a convertible.

Glass in the windows of your house blocks about 90 percent of all UV radiation. Typical office-window glass blocks around 97.5 percent of all UV radiation. A window shaded on the outside by an awning or other overhanging shade provider allows even less UV light through to the inside of a building. If you enjoy sitting indoors, at ease in your favorite chair, with warm sunshine beaming across your shoulder, keep it up. There is very little chance of skin damage.

What To Do

Be sure the windshield of your automobile is at least laminated. To boost your safety, avoid, as much as possible, sitting in an automobile in direct sunlight for extended periods of time.

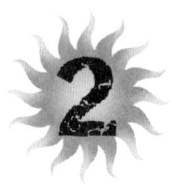

UV AND SKIN DAMAGE

IMAGINE THIS:
You noticed, just the other day, a brown patch on the skin of your shoulder, about one-fourth inch or so across. It has a ragged border, maybe—you aren't exactly sure. You picked at it, and a little blood leaked out at the edge. Should you be concerned?

KNOW YOUR SKIN TYPE

Not all skin, as you have undoubtedly noticed, is created equal. In terms of potential sun damage, the more sensitive your skin, the more careful you need to be. Types I and II face the greatest risk of developing skin cancer. Naturally dark-skinned people (types V and VI) have high concentrations of melanin, which absorbs UV radiation, so they suffer less from sunburn, skin cancer, and sun-induced aging with its subsequent wrinkling.

What To Do

The lower the number of your skin type, the greater the precautions you need to take to avoid UV radiation. Use the following chart to determine your skin type number.

Type	Characteristics	Examples
I	Very fair skin, burns easily, never tans	Blond or red hair; blue or green eyes
II	Fair skin, burns usually, tans after long hours of exposure	Blond, red, or brown hair; blue, brown, or hazel eyes
III	Medium skin, burns and tans moderately	Most Caucasians
IV	Light brown skin, burns a little, tans well	Many Asians and Hispanics
V	Dark brown skin, burns rarely, tans darkly	Many Indians and Middle Easterners
VI	Black skin, may burn with extreme exposure	Some Africans and many African Americans

DON'T GET SUNBURNED

"Alas, the sun is about as healthy as smoking cigarettes."

—Karl Neumann, MD

Ultraviolet light from the sun, striking human skin, is partly reflected, partly absorbed by outer layers, and partly transmitted to deeper layers until its energy dissipates.

UV rays will traumatize your skin when exposure time is long enough, and the result is called "sunburn." Sunburn is literally a burn caused by the sun's ultraviolet radiation (*not* its heat).

Mild and uncomplicated sunburn results in skin redness and irritation, both of which usually appear within two to six hours after exposure. The burned skin will feel hot—or at least warm—when you touch it. Redness and pain typically peak somewhere between twelve and twenty-four hours. Severe sunburn causes serious, obvious skin damage including blistering, fluid loss, and perhaps infection. Chills, fever, nausea, and vomiting may be associated with severe sunburn. Skin loss, by the way, typically occurs within four to seven days.

What To Do
Aspirin or ibuprofen, especially if started early, will help ease the pain. Cool compresses are also beneficial, and a compress soaked in half water, half milk seems to work better than just water. Cool—not ice cold—baths or showers are often useful. Aloe-based lotions, of which there are many, moisturize your burned skin, probably speed healing, and make you feel better. Drink plenty of clear fluids.

While your damaged skin heals, application of other substances—topical anesthetics, perfume, insect repellents, calamine lotion, even sunscreens—may be dangerous since your skin has increased sensitivity and increased ability to absorb substances.

Severe sunburn, with intense pain and blistering, should be seen promptly by a physician.

SLOW SKIN AGING

> "Not only can excessive solar exposure accelerate and intensify aging in skin, it can also lead to serious health risks."
> —John Browder, MD, and Betsy Beers, MD

Somewhere between the transient pain and redness of mild sunburn and the malignant cancer of melanoma (see Monitor Yourself for Malignant Melanoma) lies photoaging, the changes that occur in human skin with cumulative exposure to UV radiation. UV light, absorbed by your skin, leads to permanent damage to RNA and DNA, alterations in connective tissue, and loss of stabilization in membranes. These changes may make little or no difference in the way you function, but they can profoundly change the way you look.

Intrinsic skin changes are just a part of the natural aging process, but they are accelerated in photo-damaged skin. Extrinsic skin changes are caused by exposure to things in your environment: heat, wind, some chemicals, cigarette smoke, and, by far the most significant, UV radiation. These changes include fine and deep wrinkling, pigment alterations (including permanent spots and the red leathery skin of cutis rhomboidalis from which we get the term "redneck"), sagging, and changes in the vasculature of the skin. A form of elastosis, the breakdown of elastic fibers in your skin, is the most universal sign of photoaging. Elastosis produces a loss of elasticity. You do not see elastosis in unexposed areas of your body.

What To Do

To stop photoaging, you must stop exposing your unprotected skin to solar radiation. Use sunscreens and protective clothing, and avoid the midday sun. Although most photoaging is permanent, some changes are reversible with cessation of exposure.

BEWARE OF BASAL CELL CARCINOMA

> "The sun is responsible for over 90 percent of all skin cancers."
>
> —Skin Cancer Foundation

Skin cancer is the most common form of cancer, with more than *one million* new cases reported every year in the United States. It is the fastest growing form of cancer, over fourteen times more common than it was sixty years ago. On the plus side, if you want to call it that, it is one of the most curable forms of cancer if detected early enough. It is also preventable.

Of the three major types of skin cancer, basal cell carcinoma (BCC) ranks as the one most commonly diagnosed, with around 750,000 new cases every year. Your basal cells make up the base of your epidermis, the outer layer of skin. Too much UV radiation can cause those cells to reproduce too fast (while at the same time repressing your natural immune response to such unnatural reproduction), and a tumorous growth forms. Basal cell carcinoma usually starts as a slow-growing, small, shiny (or pearly) bump or nodule that becomes an open sore taking longer than three weeks to heal. It often bleeds, crusts over, and opens to bleed again. The cancer may be an itchy or tender reddish patch that comes and goes. Sometimes it is a pale splotch, like a scar, and sometimes a circular growth with a raised border and depressed center.

On rare occasions, these cancerous basal cells release from the tumor, usually into your blood, and take up residence in another organ, such as your liver. The cancer is said to have metastasized, and it is now a threat to your life. The survival rate of treated basal cell carcinoma, before it has a chance to metastasize, is greater than 95 percent. Unfortunately, the problem shows up again in about 40 percent of those treated.

What To Do

Check your skin often. If you suspect you have skin cancer, see your doctor as soon as possible. In the meantime, do not overexpose your unprotected skin to ultraviolet rays.

SEARCH YOURSELF FOR SQUAMOUS CELL CARCINOMA

> "Ninety percent of all skin cancers occur on parts of the body that usually aren't covered by clothing."
> —American Cancer Society

Of the three major types of skin cancer, squamous cell carcinoma (SCC) ranks as the second most common,

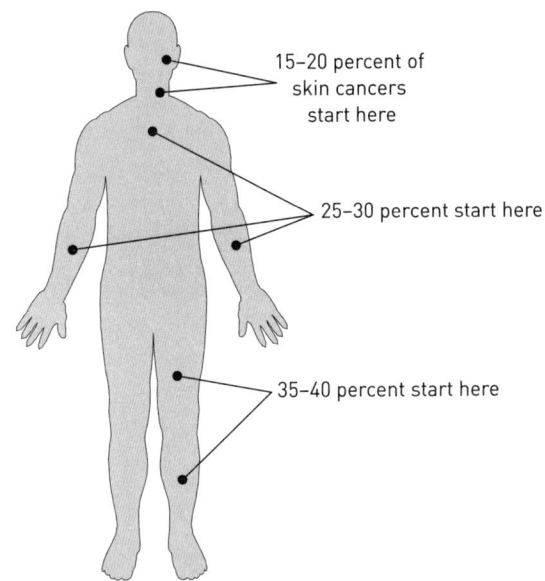

Where to check for skin cancer

Monitor your skin most carefully in the areas of the body most likely to develop cancer.

accounting for about 250,000 cases every year. Although not as common as basal cell carcinoma, its rate of increase is higher. Your squamous cells make up most of your epidermis, and they are susceptible to the same UV alterations as basal cells. This cancer may look like basal cell cancer, but it can also appear as a wart that bleeds and crusts over, bleeds and crusts over.

Cancerous squamous cells grow faster and metastasize more frequently than basal cell carcinomas, and, although generally not considered serious, these cells are more difficult to treat than basal cells if the problem is not identified early. Still, the survival rate of squamous cell carcinoma when treated before it has a chance to metastasize, is greater than 90 percent.

Common sites for any type of skin cancer are the face, ears, neck, and scalp. In the past fifty years, shoulders, backs, and chests on men, and the lower legs on women, have become increasingly common sites for skin cancer. The reason, of course, is deliberate exposure of those body parts to the sun's ultraviolet radiation.

What To Do

If you suspect you have skin cancer, see your doctor as soon as possible. In the meantime, do not overexpose your unprotected skin to ultraviolet rays. Squamous cell carcinomas may also result from overexposure to x-rays and certain chemical compounds such as coal tar, asphalt, and pitch.

MONITOR YOURSELF FOR MALIGNANT MELANOMA

> "One in five Americans and one in three Caucasians will develop skin cancer in the course of a lifetime."
> —Skin Cancer Foundation

Of the three major types of skin cancer, malignant melanoma is the least common but the most serious. With about 60,000 new cases appearing each year, melanoma currently kills more than 8000 people annually—approximately 5200 men and 2800 women. One in five people diagnosed with malignant melanoma is dead within five years. Melanomas involve your melanocytes, the cells that give your skin its color. This cancer most often originates in or near a mole, birthmark, or "beauty mark." The more moles you have, the greater your risk of melanoma. But it can also occur as a new spot and range in color from black to brown to red and blue to translucent. After they appear, they continue to grow with irregular borders.

But detected early, this cancer is cured nearly 100 percent of the time. There is about a 50 percent chance of recurrence. Instead of cumulative exposure, malignant melanoma appears more often in people who have a history of serious sunburns, especially if the sunburns occurred when they were children. If someone in your family has had this cancer, your risks are even higher. Men, as the death rate implies, and probably due to less concern over exposure to UV radiation, are diagnosed with melanoma more often than women.

Physicians employ several different techniques to remove skin cancer. The choice depends on the extent of the cancer, the position on the body, and the risks to the patient. Surgical removal accounts for 95 percent of treatments. Electrosurgery may be used, in which an electric current burns the border of the removal site to kill any remaining cancer. For people who cannot tolerate regular surgery, the cancer may be frozen and removed via a technique called cryosurgery. Another option, used

Normal Mole	Melanoma	Sign	Characteristic
		Asymmetry	Half of the mole does not match the other half.
		Border	The edges of the mole are ragged or irregular.
		Color	The color of the mole varies throughout.
		Diameter	The mole's diameter is larger than a pencil's eraser.

Photographs used by permission of the National Cancer Institute.

Melanoma, the most dangerous form of skin cancer, can be successfully treated if caught early.

most often in elderly patients, is radiation therapy, in which a beam of radiation, directed at the cancer, kills the bad cells. After it has metastasized, a melanoma usually requires chemotherapy or immunotherapy.

What To Do

The American Cancer Society recommends regularly checking yourself for the ABCD of Early Detection:

A for Asymmetry: one half of the growth does not look like the other half.

B for Border: edges are ragged, irregular, or indistinct.

C for Color: non-uniform pigmentation.

D for Diameter: any growth larger than ¼ inch (6 millimeters) should be checked.

KEEP AN EYE ON SOLAR KERATOSES

> "Regular use of sunscreens prevents the development of solar keratoses and, by implication, possibly reduces the risk of skin cancer in the long term."
> —Sandra Thompson, Damien Jolley, and Robin Marks. "Reduction of Solar Keratoses by Regular Sunscreen Use." *New England Journal of Medicine* 329, no. 16 (October 1993)

Solar keratoses, also called actinic keratoses, are growths that develop on human skin (most often the face, neck, and back of the hands) from overexposure to ultraviolet light. They are rough spots on the skin, usually in multiples, sometimes scaly and sometimes warty, sometimes skin-colored and sometimes reddish, sometimes flat and sometimes thickened. They are becoming so common some doctors suggest 50 percent of all white-skinned people over the age of forty have them, or will have them. Solar keratoses are precancerous and nonmalignant, but they are a powerful warning sign that skin cancer, probably squamous cell carcinoma, may be on the way.

Solar keratoses can be prevented in a large number of people with the regular use of sunscreens. People who already have solar keratoses sometimes see remission with the use of sunscreens. Although sunscreens are rated on their ability to prevent sunburn, not keratoses or cancer, studies show that higher SPF ratings do prevent keratoses in many people.

What To Do
- Use a sunscreen with a high SPF (at least 15) that protects against UVA and UVB every time you are exposed to ultraviolet light.
- If you develop what you think are solar keratoses, see your doctor for an evaluation. They should be treated by removal of the defective skin cells before they have a chance to degenerate into cancer.

AVOID PHOTOSENSITIVITY REACTIONS

If you are taking certain drugs for some medical conditions, using certain chemicals on your skin, or eating certain foods, you could be making yourself photosensitive, or more than normally sensitive to the sun's ultraviolet radiation. Problems of photosensitivity do not fall neatly into scientific classifications due to a wide variety of individual responses and lack of medical knowledge on the subject. But generally, photosensitivity reactions fall into three broad categories:

- Phototoxic reactions: an exaggerated normal response to sunlight, a common result of using some shampoos, perfumes, and other everyday products.
- Photoallergic reactions: an abnormal response to sunlight, usually a rash, from many medications, soaps, and cosmetics.
- Phytophotodermatitis: a reaction from getting some plant juices on your skin prior to exposure to UV light, commonly caused by lemons, limes, celery, parsley, parsnips, carrots, figs, and mustard.

A Partial List of Substances That May Cause Photosensitivity

Food additives, including cyclamates and saccharine.
Benzocaine, used in most anesthetic sprays.
Biothionol, used in some soaps and first-aid creams.
Green soap, an antimicrobial soap.
Sunscreens, especially the ones with PABA.

A Partial List of Drugs That May Cause Photosensitivity

Antidepressants, including Adapin, Asendin, Elavil, Norpramin, Vivactil.

Antihistamines, including Benadryl.

Antimicrobials, including Bactrim, Fansidar, Septra, the tetracyclines, and the doxycyclines.

Antiparasitics, including chloroquine and quinine.

Antipsychotics, including Haldol, Phenergan, Thorazine.

Diuretics, including Diamox and Lasix.

Hypoglycemics, including Diabinase, Glucotrol, Orinase, Tolinase.

NSAIDs (nonsteroidal anti-inflammatory drugs), including Clinoril, Feldene, Naprosyn, Orudis.

What To Do

Direct ultraviolet light should be avoided when you are taking a drug or using a chemical that makes you photosensitive. If you think you are having an allergic reaction, try a different brand. If you are unsure, consult your physician.

PROTECT YOUR IMMUNE SYSTEM

Natural immunity, the ability to fight off disease, can be impaired in some animals who are subjected to excesses of ultraviolet radiation. Do UV rays have that effect on humans? Yes, ultraviolet radiation, even in relatively small doses, can suppress the function of immune cells in human skin. In an Australian study, volunteers subjected to less UV light than necessary to cause mild sunburn, once daily for five days, averaged a reduction in immune cell response of 40 percent. People with dark skin experienced the same average reduction as pale-skinned people. Although these cells appear to recover four to six weeks after exposure, repeated exposure to UV radiation can lead to chronic immunosuppression. The data at this time remains inconclusive, but it is strongly suspected

VULNERABILITIES

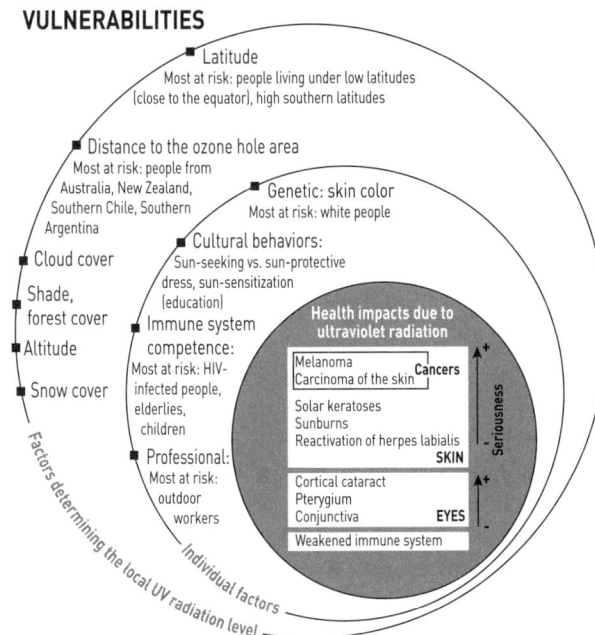

Source: World Health Organization, *Global burden of disease from solar ultraviolet radiation*, 2006.

The risk of skin cancer varies greatly from individual to individual. Know the risk to you!

that UV immunosuppression will make human skin more susceptible to skin cancers.

What To Do
Play it safe by reducing your exposure to direct sunlight.

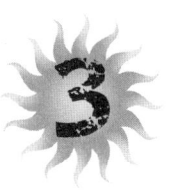

UV AND SKIN PROTECTION

IMAGINE THIS:
The heat of the sun makes you feel like you could fry an egg on your forehead, but you lathered on sunscreen with a label declaring "SPF 30." You're safe for at least three hours—right?

DO NOT TRUST WATER TO PUT OUT THE FIRE

"Approximately 80 percent of UV (radiation) penetrates 1 foot of distilled water, posing the threat of serious sunburn to scuba divers and snorkelers."
—James R. Roberts, MD, University of Cincinnati Hospital

Swimmers beware. All that water flowing with satisfying coolness over your skin does *not* protect you from UV radiation. It makes you feel safe, but, in fact, skin that has absorbed a lot of water, from about an hour of swimming, will allow UV rays to penetrate approximately four times more easily than dry skin does. Even water just on the surface of your skin, including sweat, reduces the reflectivity of light and will encourage sunburn to develop faster and deeper. The dampness of humidity plays a role in sunburn as well. You will burn faster on a hot, humid day than on a hot, dry day.

What To Do

Use a waterproof sunscreen when swimming or when exposing your skin to sunlight on a high humidity day. Use a sunscreen with a high SPF, and reapply it often—at least every two hours.

THINK TWICE BEFORE TANNING

"All tanning is visible evidence of toxic injury."
—National Institutes of Health

Genetically, you were programmed with a fixed number of melanocytes, the pigment-producing cells in your epidermis. Dark-skinned people have a lot of melanocytes while light-skinned people have few. Your number of melanocytes determines your ability to tan. The dark pigment produced by melanocytes, called melanin, causes tanning and blocks the transmission of UVB into the deeper layers of your skin.

Tanning is a two-phase phenomenon. The first phase is stimulated by UVA, involves immediate darkening of existing melanin, and lasts only a few hours. It often goes unnoticed. The second phase, stimulated by UVB, involves a lasting increase in the amount of melanin. This is a true tan. UVA, over a long period of time, will also produce a similar tan. Without repeated exposure to UV rays, tans fade over several weeks due to the constant natural loss and replacement of epidermal cells.

Tanned skin burns less easily than non-tanned skin. Quantitatively, tans provide an SPF of 2 to 4. Otherwise there are no known health benefits to tanning. And almost everyone requires at least modest sunburn in order to initiate tanning. People who tan poorly, or not at all, are at the greatest risk for developing skin cancer or other degenerative skin disorders while attempting to acquire a tan.

What To Do
The safest bet: Learn to be satisfied with the natural shade of your skin.

UNDERSTAND SPF
Until recently, SPF stood for Sun Protection Factor. It now stands for Sunburn Protection Factor due to changes demanded by the Food and Drug Administration (see Understand the *New* UVA Rating System).

SPF tells you how long you can be exposed to sunlight before you burn, compared to exposure time without a sunscreen. The SPF rating system allows sunscreens to be rated from 2 to 50+. If your unprotected skin starts turning red with twenty minutes of exposure, SPF 15 will give you, theoretically, fifteen times that amount of time—around five hours—before you start turning red. SPF may also be thought of as a percentage: SPF 15 protects against approximately 93 percent of UVB radiation, SPF 30 protects against about 97 percent, and SPF 50 against about 99 percent.

And, remember, SPF relates *only to UVB radiation*.

Although it seems that SPF 15 would do for almost anyone, studies show that higher SPF ratings offer greater protection, especially during the first minutes of exposure to UV radiation. This fact could be especially important to people with sensitive skin (see Know Your Skin Type).

Keep in mind there are problems with SPF ratings. For one thing, sunscreens, whatever the SPF rating, lose most of their effectiveness after two hours, requiring reapplication. And for another thing, "turning red" is only one indication of skin damage. The damage done by UVA is not necessarily related to burning.

What To Do
+ Most adults should choose an SPF of at least 15 if they want to tan and SPF 25 if they want to prevent, or at least reduce, tanning.
+ If you are fair skinned or anticipate exposure for an extended period of time, always choose an SPF higher than 15.
+ Because childhood sunburns increase the risk of skin cancer later in life, children should use an SPF of at least 25 starting at approximately six months of age. (Keep children less than six months of age out of direct sunlight. See Do Not Mix Babies and Bright Sunlight.)

UNDERSTAND THE *NEW* UVA RATING SYSTEM
Despite the fact that labels on sunscreen often say you are protected against UVA radiation, there has been no

common system for testing for UVA protection—until now. Along with a new FDA-mandated testing system, there is a new UVA rating system, a four-star system with one star indicating low protection and four stars indicating maximum UVA protection. The UVA rating system, like the SPF rating system, provides a validated method for measuring sun protection. You will find the UVA rating near the SPF rating on labels of sunscreens.

Labels must also include the following warning: "UV exposure from the sun increases the risk of skin cancer, premature skin aging, and other skin damage. It is important to decrease UV exposure by limiting time in the sun, wearing protective clothing, and using sunscreen."

Furthermore, products without UVA protection are required to include on the label these words: "No UVA protection."

However, these changes were not required to appear on sunscreen labels until around May 2009.

What To Do

Contact sunscreen manufacturers and encourage them to adopt the new testing, ratings, and labeling for UVA protection as soon as possible. In the meantime, choose name brands of sunscreen since those products have a better chance of being labeled correctly.

USE SUNSCREEN

Sunscreens contain chemicals that stop UV radiation from reaching your skin. To qualify as a sunscreen, a product must have an SPF of at least 2 (see Understand SPF). The best products have at least three active ingredients that work against UVB *and* UVA radiation.

Sunscreens are formulated with bases of lotion, cream, gel, oil, or wax. There is no UV protective benefit to a specific base. The choice is personal, usually determined by which one feels best to you. Some bases, however, move around on your skin or off your skin more quickly via heat, sweat, and water. Some experts refer to the movement of sunscreen bases as the "migratory factor."

Some sunscreens, depending on the base, are labeled "water-resistant" or "waterproof." Water resistance implies the product will work for approximately forty-five minutes of swimming or heavy sweating. Waterproof sunscreens should be working after eighty minutes under the same conditions.

SUNSCREEN UPDATE:
A new sunscreen ingredient, ecamsule, promises greater protection from UVA than ever before. But ecamsule's peak protection stops at about 344 nm. Since UVA wavelengths reach 400 nm, some UVA will still be able to penetrate your skin, no matter how great the protection of sunscreen. How important is this fact? No one knows yet.

What To Do
+ Read the label carefully, and choose a sunscreen that at least promises maximum protection against UVA and UVB radiation.

- Choose a sunscreen with a base that resists "migration."
- Before coating your body with a sunscreen, apply it to a small area, about the size of your hand, and wait an hour to see if you develop a rash or other skin irritation that indicates you are allergic to that particular sunscreen. If you are allergic, try a different brand.
- If you are swimming or sweating a lot or if you have especially oily skin, use a water-resistant or waterproof sunscreen.
- If you are taking a medication, check with your doctor or pharmacist concerning possible side effects with sunscreens or sunlight.

APPLY SUNSCREENS CORRECTLY

> "The only two realistic solutions to prevention of overexposure to solar radiation are limitation of exposure time and use of effective sunscreens."
> —James R. Roberts, MD

SPF is based on a uniform sunscreen covering of your skin of approximately 2 milligrams per square centimeter. If you are not uniformly coated, you are not uniformly protected. The average adult wearing an average swimsuit (males: boxer-short size; females: one piece) should use an average of one ounce (30 cc) of sunscreen for one application, approximately the amount needed to fill a shot glass. Proper application is arguably the single most important factor in determining the effectiveness of your sunscreen.

What To Do

- For best results, apply sunscreen when your skin is dry. Moisture mixes with the product and reduces its effectiveness.
- Apply a sunscreen at least thirty minutes before exposure to sunlight to allow it to be absorbed and to dry on your skin.
- Reapply sunscreens often, at least every two hours, during periods of exposure.
- Do not just smear it on—rub it in.
- Have someone help you apply sunscreen to hard-to-reach areas such as the middle of your back.
- Be especially careful to apply a thick coating to areas where skin damage shows up often, such as the nose, tops of ears, behind the ears.
- Do not forget the part in your hair and bald spots.

BLOCK THE SUN

Some opaque creams and pastes totally block all UV radiation. In fact, when properly applied, they block all light from reaching your skin. Although some sunscreens with high SPF ratings are referred to as blocks (those with an SPF rating of 12 or higher), only substances that prevent all light from reaching your skin are true sunblocks. Zinc oxide, titanium dioxide, and red veterinary petrolatum are common ingredients in sunblocks. They do not carry an SPF number and do not irritate skin because they are not absorbed into the skin. They offer excellent protection from the sun.

Because sunblocks are often messy, greasy, and

generally considered unappealing, many people choose not to use them. Some products, however, are offered in designer colors to match the frames of your sunglasses or your swimsuit—in case that matters to you.

Other substances can be used as sunblocks if commercially manufactured products are unavailable: ashes from a fire, charcoal, mud or clay mixed into a paste, axle grease. Your "unappeal factor," however, will go way up.

What To Do
+ Apply sunblocks thickly, so that none of your skin shows through, similar to the way a clown applies makeup.
+ Apply sunblocks on your nose, lips, the tops of your ears, or other sensitive areas, where exposure tends to be highest.
+ Use a sunblock if you are especially sensitive to sunscreens.

DON'T GIVE THE SUN ANY LIP
Human lips are a favorite place for skin damage to appear later in life. For one thing, the skin on lips is very thin. For another thing, lips have very little melanin. Lips are a favorite place for you to forget to apply sunscreen, or to apply sunscreen too thin because it does not taste very good. Even when applied appropriately, sunscreen comes off your lips faster than any other body part due to lip licking, lip wiping, eating, and drinking. The lips of women suffer far less sun damage than the lips of men, and the

reason may be apparent: Women tend to cover their lips with products—lipsticks and lip balms—far more often than men.

Sun damage to lips may appear as a freckly, scaly, pinkish growth on your lips. If it goes away in a week or so, you are probably okay. If it becomes sore or painful, refuses to heal, changes color, or grows in size, check in with your doctor.

What To Do
Buy a lip balm or lip sunscreen with an SPF of at least 15, with 25 being even better. Use it often while your lips are exposed to UV radiation. The taste of many lip balms, by the way, is acceptable to most people.

DRESS FOR THE SUN: PART 1
Even though long-sleeved shirts and long pants offer more protection than shorts and T-shirts, you may not be getting the amount of skin damage control you want from your clothing. UPF stands for Ultraviolet Protection Factor, and it tells you how much UV light is absorbed by your clothing. As with SPF, UPF is a number based on how well a fabric absorbs or reflects UV radiation. A fabric with a UPF of 10 allows only about one-tenth of UV light to pass through and reach your skin. Donning a white T-shirt under direct sunlight gives you an average UPF of 7, while a long-sleeved, dark-colored denim shirt can provide a UPF of 1700 (which means UV light is completely blocked).

Some emerging manufacturers specialize in clothing that is loose and comfortable with both the fibers and the weaving method chosen for maximum UV protection. With special UV protective clothing, you may find yourself spending more money than you intended, but you will find yourself comfortable and well protected from UV radiation.

What To Do

Consider special clothing manufactured to keep 97–98.5 percent of UV radiation from reaching your skin.

DRESS FOR THE SUN: PART 2

Ultraviolet light can reach your skin in varying degrees through the clothing you choose to wear, depending not only on how much of your skin is covered but also on the tightness of the weave, the fit of the clothing, the color, the amount of moisture in the clothing, and the type of material.

What To Do

- Hold your clothing up to a bright light. The more light showing through, the more ultraviolet radiation is getting through. The clothing you wear during extended periods of exposure to direct sunlight should have a tight weave.
- Wear clothing that fits loosely. When clothing is stretched over part of your body, the UV protection is reduced, sometimes dramatically. One garment, say a shirt, can be three or four times more protective at your waist than it is where it stretches over your shoulder.

- Wear dark clothing. Dyed fabric, in general, blocks more UV light than undyed fabric. A green T-shirt, for instance, will provide approximately 30 percent more UV protection than a white cotton T-shirt.
- Consider the fabric. Tightly woven cotton tends to offer more protection than tightly woven polyesters. A pair of blue denim jeans can provide 200 times more protection than a loosely woven nylon shirt.
- Keep your clothing dry. No matter the weave or color or material, water, including sweat, enhances the transparency of any garment. A T-shirt can lose up to one half its ability to protect you when it is wet.

WEAR THE RIGHT HAT

> "Anything shorter than three inches isn't very effective."
>
> —Madhu Pathak, PhD, dermatologist,
> Harvard Medical School

Basal cell carcinoma, remember, appears most often on the face, ears, and neck—and the right hat can do much to protect those areas, as well as providing protection for your eyes. Baseball caps, even caps with extra long front brims, protect much of your face—which, of course, is good—but still allow the sun to reach your ears and neck.

What To Do

Three inches of brim on your hat, all the way around, is required to provide enough shade to prevent skin damage.

Up to 85 percent of direct UV light can be blocked with a wide, circumferential brim. For some reason, probably due to greater light dispersion, floppy brims offer a little more protection than rigid brims.

An option is a commercially made, front-brimmed cap with a French Foreign Legion–type flap sewn on the back to protect your neck and ears. You can also make your own, or you can make do in a pinch by placing a bandanna or other piece of cloth under your baseball cap with most of the cloth hanging down over your neck and ears.

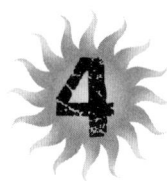

UV AND EYE PROTECTION

IMAGINE THIS:
Bright sunlight makes it impossible to do anything but squint without sunglasses. But you're wearing sunglasses. They were cheap, but the lenses are as black as coal, so your eyes are safe from sun damage—aren't they?

WEAR SUNGLASSES: PREVENT SOLAR RETINITIS

"Since the time of Plato, visual disturbances have been associated with sun viewing."
—"Solar Retinopathy," American Ophthalmological Society

Your retina, the innermost part of your eye, the part that receives images directly from the lens of your eye, is your immediate instrument of vision. Any inflamed condition of the retina is called retinitis. Although solar retinitis most often results in people who have stared too long at an eclipse of the sun, an increasing number of cases are being reported in patients who have been merely sunbathing or exercising in direct sunlight during periods of reduced ozone concentration. What happens is this: Your eye's lens, working much like a magnifying glass, focuses solar radiation on your retina and burns it.

Those people affected usually have normal vision or better than normal vision, but soon after exposure to the sun, signs of eye damage develop that include reduced ability to see, a blind spot in the field of vision, an intolerance for bright light, and seeing unusual colors or shapes. Some people who develop solar retinitis never fully recover, but most sufferers regain normal eyesight within three to nine months.

What To Do

Wear sunglasses that protect your eyes from solar radiation (see Wear Sunglasses!).

WEAR SUNGLASSES: PREVENT CATARACTS

Cataracts are opacities (like a cloudy film) of the lens of the human eye, or the capsule of the lens, or both. As cataracts develop, your ability to see diminishes and finally goes away. Surgery can often restore sight, with the use of eyeglasses. Not long ago, cataracts were considered an unavoidable result of aging, but it is now believed they can be postponed, even prevented. The three main contributors to cataracts, other than aging, are cigarette smoking, a diet poor in vitamins C and E, beta carotene, and other antioxidants . . . and lifelong exposure to ultraviolet light.

Dark-skinned people are less likely to develop skin cancer, but dark-eyed people are more likely to develop cataracts from UV rays than blue-, green-, and gray-eyed people. The reason probably lies in the fact that dark eyes have more melanin, and melanin absorbs more solar radiation, and over time, more damage is done to the lens of the eye.

What To Do

Choose sunglasses that protect your eyes from all UV rays, from at least 75 percent of visible light, and from violet/blue light (which may further degenerate the retina). Wide-brimmed hats add further protection for your eyes. And remember: The darker your eyes, the more important your choice of sunglasses.

WEAR SUNGLASSES: PREVENT SNOW BLINDNESS

The cornea of your eye can sunburn, a problem called ultraviolet keratitis or photokeratitis, or more commonly, snow blindness. It occurs most often on bright, snow-covered days, and thus the common name. You may remember that clean snow can reflect up to 85 percent of UV radiation back to your face (see Avoid a Reflection on You), so your eyes are bombarded with direct UV light and reflected UV light when you are outside on a blanket of cold and white. Although UVA could be part of the problem, it is probably UVB that does most of the damage in cases of snow blindness. And even on snow under cloudy skies, you may also remember, your eyes are at risk.

In an hour of high-level exposure, or a few hours on bright days at less than high-level exposure, the damage can be done, but it is usually six to twelve hours before the appearance of the signs and symptoms of snow blindness—the pain, feeling like sand is in your eyes; the sensitivity to light that makes it difficult, or impossible, to use your eyes (the "blindness"); a flow of tears; red eyes; and sometimes eyelid swelling. Spontaneous healing, on the plus side, usually occurs within twenty-four hours, but repeated snow blindness can cause yellowing of the lens of your eye and cataracts.

What To Do

If you are snow blind, reducing your pain is the main goal. Flushing eyes gently with cold water or cold compresses on the eyes will help. Anti-inflammatory drugs such as aspirin and ibuprofen may help. You may ask your doctor for a topical ophthalmic anesthetic (painkilling eye ointment) or a prescription-strength painkilling drug. Patch the eyes to protect them from light. Or you can grin and bear it. If you are not significantly better in twenty-four hours, see your doctor for sure.

Snow blindness is entirely preventable. Wear sunglasses that protect your eyes from UV light. The sunglasses should wrap around or, even better, have side shields to protect your eyes from reflected light.

WEAR SUNGLASSES!

Ultraviolet light is either filtered out or absorbed by your sunglasses, depending on the lens material, thickness of the lens, and the way the lens is processed. Both plastic and glass lenses can have absorptive tints added for maximum UV protection. For glass, tints are usually added during the early stages of manufacture. These tints are melted into the glass and are permanent. For plastic, the tints are added late in the manufacturing process. These tints adhere by surface absorption into the plastic, and being organic compounds, they may fade over time. Tints come in many colors and range from dark to light. Both plastic and glass can have absorptive coatings added after manufacture. They stick better to glass, but these surface coatings can be scratched off of both glass and plastic.

What To Do

Wear good sunglasses. How do you know if your sunglasses are good? Unfortunately, it is not as easy as you may think. The darkness of the lens, for instance, is not an indicator of the UV protection. Inadequately treated dark lenses can actually be harmful, offering little protection while keeping your pupils open to long-term damage. Labels on name brands that guarantee protection can usually be trusted (see Understand Labels on Sunglasses). Labels on imported brands are sometimes worth no more than the paper—or plastic—they are printed on. Your safest bet is to have the effectiveness of your sunglasses checked with a spectrophotometer by your local optometrist or ophthalmologist (see Test Your Sunglasses).

Sunglasses also need to fit properly, resting on your nose, not on your cheeks. The lens should come as close to your eyes as possible without letting your eyelashes touch the plastic or glass.

Avoid sunglasses that cause image distortion, which can lead to eyestrain and headaches. Wraparound lenses are especially susceptible to peripheral distortion. For nonprescription lenses, hold your sunglasses at arm's length and look at a straight line (a doorway, for example). If the straight line is bent through your sunglasses, your sight is being optically distorted.

UNDERSTAND LABELS ON SUNGLASSES

Shopping for a pair of sunglasses that will properly protect your eyes, as mentioned earlier, is not always easy. Many inexpensive glasses, remember, are not labeled or are incorrectly labeled. In other words, even if the label says you are protected, you may not be getting as much protection against UVB and UVA as you think. Here is why: The current FDA standards require only voluntary, not mandatory, compliance by the manufacturers of sunglasses. However, if you purchase a recognized brand of sunglasses, and if the manufacturer has labeled the sunglasses as to UV protection, you will almost always be getting the eye protection the label says you will get. You will almost always pay more, too.

Labels on quality sunglasses should also tell you the amount of visible light allowed through the lens. Standard sunglasses allow the transmission of an average of 15–25 percent of visible light, which is enough to provide comfort in most conditions. However, you may want less visible light transmission in some conditions such as bright sunlight reflected from clean snow. And note that sunglasses that let only 8 percent of visible light through do not allow you to see well enough to drive in most conditions.

What To Do

Look for sunglasses from reputable manufacturers and with a label that claims to protect your eyes from at least 98 percent of UVA and UVB. If you want eye comfort in intense light conditions, choose sunglasses that transmit only 5–10 percent of visible light. And to be absolutely sure, have your sunglasses tested (see Test Your Sunglasses).

TEST YOUR SUNGLASSES

You either already knew or you now know that UV light is invisible, and that you cannot tell how effective your sunglasses are by looking at the tint of the lenses. Just because the lenses are dark, in other words, does not mean they are protecting your eyes from UV radiation. Continued use of poor-quality sunglasses, of course, can do serious damage to your eyes.

If you are using sunglasses purchased several years ago, or are wearing prescription sunglasses, you may have no idea as to how effective they are at screening out the sun's UV rays. However, buying new sunglasses—especially ones with prescription lenses—is expensive, so you do not want to throw away glasses that are working properly.

What To Do

Take your sunglasses into an optometrist or optical shop that can test them for UV protection with a spectrophotometer.

(A spectrophotometer is actually two instruments: a spectrometer that produces light and a photometer that measures the intensity of light.) There may be no charge for this service. If your existing prescription sunglasses are not blocking UV effectively, you can have the lenses treated with a special coating to block nearly 100 percent of UV light. This is a less expensive option than ordering a new set of glasses.

CONSIDER PRESCRIPTION SUNGLASSES

If you need prescription lenses to adjust your eyesight, and if you need sunglasses at the same time, you have two choices:

You can get your prescription glasses with photochromic lenses. First introduced by Corning Glass Works in 1964, photochromic lenses have silver and chloride ions included in the glass when it is formed. When exposed to ultraviolet or blue light, the ions dissociate and cluster into specks that absorb, usually, 100 percent of UVB and 93–98 percent of UVA radiation. The more light hitting the lens, the darker it grows. Some photochromic lenses are also temperature sensitive, growing darker in cold air and lighter in warm air.

You can buy prescription sunglasses—optics with permanent tints, already treated for protection against UV rays. Many companies offer a wide variety of prescription sport optics, glasses designed with specific sports in mind, such as skiing, biking, and fishing. Note also that some contact lenses are manufactured with UV protection.

What To Do

Do not fail to wear sunglasses if you need prescription glasses. In the United States, some states require all prescription sunglasses to be purchased from a licensed optical dispenser, in which case you have to visit your optician, while some states allow you to place orders directly from manufacturers. Either way, they are available.

CONSIDER OVERGLASSES

If you wear prescription glasses, you certainly are aware by now that you face special problems in protecting your eyes from intense sunlight. With today's higher UV levels, you may also often need eyewear with side protection. Up to 40 percent of UV radiation can enter your eyes from the sides and tops of conventional prescription sunglasses.

The category of eyewear termed "overglasses" includes any large, protective shield that surrounds your eyes. Ski goggles, for instance, large enough to wear over prescription glasses are overglasses. Of particular concern here are UV protective overglasses designed to fit comfortably—and stylishly, some people might think— over existing eyewear. The sides of these glasses are made of the same polycarbonate material used for the lenses, so peripheral vision is preserved, making them suitable for driving. The glasses come in a variety of tints and frame colors. Some models offer polarized lenses (lenses that eliminate glare), while others block blue-violet light as well as UVB and UVA.

What To Do
If you are interested, talk to your optometrist about overglasses.

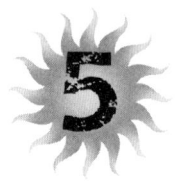

UV: MORE GOOD THINGS TO DO

IMAGINE THIS:
You are hiking along a beach, near the ebb and flow of the sea, and the wide umbrella you carry creates a patch of shade that reaches down to your toes. With all the protection you're beneath, you can save the sunscreen for another day—okay?

BE VACATION-WISE

Vacations! Time to break away for some rest, relaxation, and recreation. Time for some fresh air and sunshine—but not too much sunshine!

Before packing the car or booking that plane ticket, consider how the choice of date and location affects your exposure to ultraviolet radiation. You can reduce your risk of sunburn—and skin cancer—by picking your vacation time or vacation spot thoughtfully. Here are some examples, using the UV Index at the National Weather Service Climate Prediction Center (www.cpc.ncep.noaa.gov).

Heading for Florida and some beach time in the Keys—and spring break, around March 20, looks good.

But a peek at the UV history of Miami shows a mean UV Index of 8 around that time, high and dangerous. However, if you visit the Florida Keys around January 20, only two months earlier, the mean UV Index is 4, and you will be exposed to only 50 percent as much UV radiation.

Or how about a ski vacation, sometime in spring, and the first week of April looks good for you. How about the Colorado Rockies? Can the Index help you decide? Here are some means from the UV Index of four ski areas for early April:

Aspen, Colorado	6
Salt Lake City, Utah	5
Jackson Hole, Wyoming	5
Bozeman, Montana	4

You will probably receive less exposure to UV radiation skiing in Utah or Wyoming than in Colorado—and one-third less exposure to UV radiation skiing in Montana.

What To Do

To minimize UV exposure on your next vacation, check the UV Index for several appealing destinations—and consider the safest destination.

DO NOT MIX BABIES AND BRIGHT SUNLIGHT

The delicate skin of infants—one year of age and younger—is especially sensitive to bright and direct sunlight. Their immature immune systems are more at risk (see Protect Your Immune System), and one deep and extensive sunburn during childhood can double your child's risk of skin cancer later in life.

The use of sunscreens on infants remains controversial. It potentially increases their body core temperature, if lathered on thick and extensively, increasing the risk of overheating. The strong chemicals in some sunscreens can also irritate an infant's skin. Most experts, to be safe, do *not* recommend applying sunscreens to babies less than six months old and only sparingly, if at all, to infants between six months and one year.

Infants—and children under ten—are also more susceptible to irreversible eye damage from UV light due to the transmissibility of the lens (more bad light, in other words, gets to their retinas).

What To Do
- Do not expose infants to direct sunlight. Keep them in shade. Use covered strollers and large umbrellas.
- Do not use sunscreens on infants of six months or less. On older infants, if you choose to use a sunscreen, pick one that contains inert zinc oxide instead of the stronger chemicals. Many companies now make sunscreens just for babies and young children. The first time you use a brand, apply it first to a small area, about the size of the infant's hand, and wait a half hour to see if there is a skin reaction. Never use baby oil as sun protection.
- Buy your children their own sunglasses, and wear yours as an example. Several manufacturers make sunglasses especially for really small people.

TEACH YOUR CHILDREN WELL

A myth has persisted for many years, and it goes like this: 80 percent of sun exposure occurs by the age of eighteen—so there is nothing we can do if we are older. Not so. By age eighteen, we have been bombarded with less than 25 percent of our total lifetime sun exposure. (It is, in fact, men over forty who are currently getting the highest annual amount of UV rays.)

But this is also true: *Children are more susceptible to environmental threats than adults.* Children are not little adults. Direct sunlight is even worse for children than it is for grown-ups. Kids burn faster, and cumulative skin damage starts with the first exposure. Intense, one-day exposure during a child's lifetime, say a day at the beach unprotected, may be more harmful than numerous short-term exposures. But the damage may not show up for thirty years. And the eyes of children aged ten and younger, as mentioned earlier, allow more damaging light through than adult eyes do—and damage may occur with the first intense exposure.

What To Do
- Be a role model.
- Use protective clothing, a hat, and sunglasses on your children. Blocking the sun from reaching their skin is the safest solution.
- Teach your children to use sunscreen. Choose sunscreen with SPF 15 or higher. For young children, products with a milky lotion or cream base feel better to their skin, do not contain alcohol which can sting,

and are easier to see where applied compared to clear lotions. Sunscreens should be applied carefully, covering all exposed skin, especially the nose, ears, lower face, and neck, but avoiding the upper and lower eyelids. Kids tend to rub sunscreen into their eyes; not all screens are eye-irritating, but many are.
+ Teach your children to wear a hat to protect their upper faces.
+ Teach your children to wear sunglasses.

USE A UV METER

For up-to-the-moment data on how much UV radiation is striking you, products are available. The information they provide is not precise, but it is dependable. One product is a card, and the other is a small monitoring device (both can be found through an online search).

The card is about the size of a credit card, low-cost and reusable, known as a UV card or UV sensometer. It looks, in fact, like a plastic credit card, but instead of a magnetic strip, it has a strip with a UV-sensitive chemical that changes color. You simply hold the card up to the sun for about twenty seconds, and the white strip changes color to indicate the UV intensity—darker shades of purple indicating stronger UV levels. The cards are coded to help you estimate the amount of UV radiation you are receiving. (To make another reading, you will need to cover the card or keep it indoors for several minutes to let it turn white again.) The device can also be useful for testing the effectiveness of your sunglasses and your sunscreen. If you put the card behind the lenses of your sunglasses, it should remain white if the glasses block 100 percent of UV rays. Smearing sunscreen over the strip and then exposing it to sunlight will give you an idea of how well that particular product is working. Another good experiment is to compare the intensity of UV rays at midday with levels later in the evening at your location. You can also use the device to convince yourself that UV radiation is still present on cloudy days.

Several brands of monitors are available. They are compact, fitting easily into a pocket, and, although more expensive than a card, costs are surprisingly low. Some allow you to adjust the device to your skin type, and all of them give a ballpark number indicating the amount of UV light currently hitting your skin. The information shows up on an LED indicator. Some models sound a warning when the amount of UV radiation reaches high levels.

What To Do
If you want pinpoint accuracy, you will not find it in either device—but every little bit of help in saving your skin is worth considering.

CREATE MORE SHADE IN YOUR BACKYARD
As ozone levels drop, you may want to develop more shady areas for your own yard. You and your family can still enjoy being outside while being protected from excessive UV rays. Adding shade can be accomplished by landscaping (planting more trees) and by "home improvement" projects that involve the construction of covers or canopies over decks and patio areas.

What To Do

When planning these projects, keep in mind the angle and path of both the summer sun and winter sun. What you want are trees and structures that deliver maximum shade during the summer months but are designed and placed in such a way as to provide warm and mild sunlight during the winter. Planting deciduous trees on the south side of your house is one way to do this. During summer they will give you welcome shade when you need it, and in the fall, they will drop their leaves, permitting the winter sun to brighten your windows and help lower your heating bill.

Deck and patio areas should be covered with high roofs open on the sides for summer ventilation. Deck and patio floors should be stained or painted a dark color or constructed of nonreflective material. Screens that keep out bugs help keep out some UV radiation, the amount variable.

USE PORTABLE SHADE

Sun umbrellas, or parasols, are not a new idea. The word *parasol*, in fact, comes from the French and means "to ward off the sun." You will be cooler under an umbrella of reflective silver as opposed to heat-absorbing black. While you can use an ordinary umbrella to provide modest protection, the ideal parasol should be made out of a fabric that effectively stops UV rays (see Dress for the Sun: Part 1). Such products are available from manufacturers that promise a UPF of 50 and a 98 percent blockage of UV rays.

What To Do

Using a sun umbrella is a good idea, whether you are hiking in the desert or hanging around the beach. But remember: parasols and beach umbrellas do *not* prevent skin damage from reflected UV radiation. You should still be wearing sunscreen on exposed skin.

BOOT THE BOOTH

> "Tanning booths damage your skin just like real sunlight does."
> —American Academy of Family Physicians website (www.aafp.org, accessed January 2008)

According to manufacturers of tanning booths and sunlamps and operators of tanning salons, you can get an artificially induced tan from light sources that emit mainly UVA radiation, which is true. And artificially induced tans from booths are indistinguishable from sun-induced tans. However, you should have concerns about tanning salons: There are no controls to guarantee the light sources are what they claim to be, and UVA rays, which penetrate deeper into your skin than UVB, are now known to be unsafe. UVA, as mentioned earlier, prematurely ages skin, probably promotes cataracts, induces phototoxic reactions more often than UVB, and augments the cancer-causing effects of UVB. For those reasons, the American Academy of Dermatology discourages the use of artificial UV sources for cosmetic purposes. The Federal Drug Administration (FDA) estimates, furthermore, that a half hour under a sunlamp can be as detrimental as a half hour on the beach at midday.

What To Do
Do not think tanning booths and sunlamps are safe alternatives to direct sunlight.

CONSUME ENOUGH BETA-CAROTENE AND VITAMINS C AND E

Free radicals are unstable molecules created by your body by several normal chemical processes. Creation of free radicals gets a boost by some environmental influences including cigarette smoke and solar radiation. Being "incomplete" chemically, free radicals take pieces of other molecules, causing the production of abnormal compounds that probably play a role in the development of cancer and other diseases.

Beta-carotene (a member of a large group of nutrients called carotenoids) and Vitamins C and E are antioxidants. Antioxidants are substances with the unique property of being willing and able to destroy free radicals. Do they help prevent cancer? Nobody knows for sure, but everyone agrees your body needs an adequate supply of all nutrients to stay healthy—and antioxidants might help prevent cancer.

How much do you need? For decades the Institute of Medicine of the National Academies has maintained the Recommended Daily Allowance (RDA) of nutrients. The RDA for vitamin C is 75 milligrams for women and 90 milligrams for men. Eating more vitamin C than you need is relatively harmless since the vitamin is water-soluble, and your body excretes what it can't use. For vitamin E the RDA is 15 milligrams. Vitamin E is fat-soluble, your body stores it, and too much can become toxic. Nobody knows exactly where vitamin E toxicity begins. There is no RDA for beta-carotene, but experts generally recommend 150–180 milligrams a day.

What To Do

Your best bet is to eat plenty of healthy food. Consume at least five servings of fruit and vegetables every day. Antioxidant-rich foods are typically colorful: orange, yellow, and dark green.

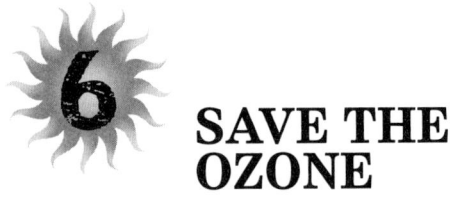

SAVE THE OZONE

IMAGINE THIS:
You read that the production of ozone-destroying chlorofluorocarbons (CFCs) was phased out about ten years ago. The ozone shield is well on its way to being repaired, and you can relax—can't you?

DO NOT BUY OZONE-EATING CHEMICALS

Steps have been taken that will help save our ozone shield. The production and importation of virgin halon, for example, has been banned in the United States (but some recycled halon is allowed). Some CFCs, especially refrigerants, are currently being recovered and recycled instead of being released into the air. Ozone-destroying products, however, remain on store shelves today.

Here is a partial list of products that potentially damage our ozone shield:

+ Halon fire extinguishers
+ Cars that still use R-12 Freon in the air conditioner
+ Do-it-yourself pressure cans of R-12 to put in car air conditioners
+ Boat horns, VCR-head cleaners, electronics cleaning sprays that contain CFCs

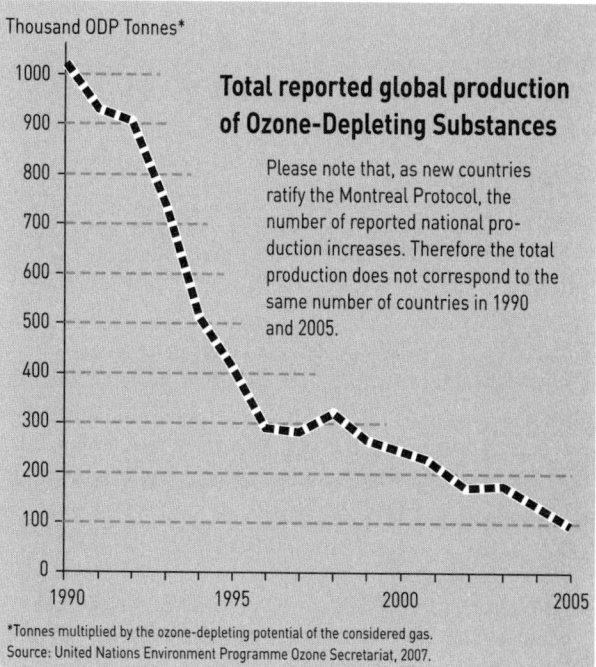

*Tonnes multiplied by the ozone-depleting potential of the considered gas.
Source: United Nations Environment Programme Ozone Secretariat, 2007.

The recognition of the dangers of ozone-depleting chemicals has caused an unprecedented worldwide reduction in the production of such chemicals.

+ Rigid plastic foam products—cups, plates, building insulation—that are not made CFC-free
+ Household products that contain ozone-eating chemicals such as fabric protectors, stain removers, solvents, and many pesticides

What To Do

While politicians and chemical company executives squabble over phase-out timetables, you can vote with your wallet today. For your safety and the safety of future generations, please do not buy products that contain CFCs, HCFCs, halons, carbon tetrachloride, methyl bromide, or methyl chloroform (sometimes called 1,1,1 trichloro-ethylene). Read the labels on chemical containers *before* you buy.

HELP RECLAIM OZONE-DEPLETING CHEMICALS

Ozone-depleting chemicals, as a result of new laws and the adoption of substitute chemicals, are slowly disappearing but often are recoverable and recyclable. You can help by making sure that the chemicals in existing products are reclaimed whenever possible.

What To Do

- Be sure your vehicle's air conditioner is serviced at a repair shop that uses equipment to remove CFCs, and that they return these CFCs for safe disposal or recycling. Do not junk an old car without first removing the Freon from the air conditioner.
- Take similar actions when servicing or disposing of refrigerators and air conditioner units. It is not legal to simply dump an old air conditioner, freezer, or refrigerator. Call your city or county government or call the Environmental Protection Agency (EPA) ozone information hotline at 800-296-1996 or www.epa.gov.

- Do not throw your halon fire extinguishers in the trash. Find out how to recycle halon from the Halon Recycling Corporation at 800-258-1283 or www.halon.org.

Thank you!

APPENDICES

THE TEN UV PROTECTION ESSENTIALS
1. Stay UV aware
2. Wear an adequate hat
3. Wear protective clothing
4. Wear effective sunglasses
5. Use effective sunscreen properly
6. Use effective lip balm
7. Eat a diet rich in antioxidants
8. Enjoy the shade
9. Get regular checkups for skin cancer
10. Don't get sunburned

RESOURCES
Auerbach, Paul, ed. *Wilderness Medicine*, 4th ed. St. Louis: Mosby, 2001.
All About Vision at www.allaboutvision.com
American Academy of Dermatology at www.aad.org
American Academy of Optometry at www.aaopt.org
American Academy of Pediatrics at www.aap.org
American Cancer Society at www.cancer.org
American Melanoma Foundation at www.melanomafoundation.org
American Ophthalmological Society at www.aosonline.org
Centers for Disease Control at www.cdc.gov
Dermatology Consultants at www.dermconsultants.com
Environmental Protection Agency (EPA) at www.epa.gov

Eyecare Trust at www.eye-care.org.uk

Feather River Air Quality Management District at www.fraqmd.org

Institute of Medicine of the National Academies at www.iom.edu

Mayo Clinic at www.mayoclinic.com

NASA Ozone Hole Watch at http://ozonewatch.gsfc.nasa.gov

National Cancer Institute at www.cancer.gov

National Eye Institute at www.nei.nih.gov

National Institutes of Health (NIH) at www.nih.gov

National Oceanic and Atmospheric Administration (NOAA) at www.nws.noaa.gov

National Weather Service Climate Prediction Center at www.cpc.ncep.noaa.gov

Skin Cancer Foundation at www.skincancer.org

Sun Protection Australia at www.sunprotection.com.au

SunSmart of Australia at www.sunsmart.com.au

U.S. Food and Drug Administration (FDA) at www.fda.gov

World Health Organization (WHO) at www.who.int

THE MOUNTAINEERS, founded in 1906, is a nonprofit outdoor activity and conservation club, whose mission is "to explore, study, preserve, and enjoy the natural beauty of the outdoors...." Based in Seattle, Washington, the club is now one of the largest such organizations in the United States, with seven branches throughout Washington State.

The Mountaineers sponsors both classes and year-round outdoor activities in the Pacific Northwest, which include hiking, mountain climbing, ski-touring, snowshoeing, bicycling, camping, kayaking and canoeing, nature study, sailing, and adventure travel. The club's conservation division supports environmental causes through educational activities, sponsoring legislation, and presenting informational programs. All club activities are led by skilled, experienced volunteers, who are dedicated to promoting safe and responsible enjoyment and preservation of the outdoors.

If you would like to participate in these organized outdoor activities or the club's programs, consider a membership in The Mountaineers. For information and an application, write or call The Mountaineers, Club Headquarters, 7700 Sand Point Way NE, Seattle, WA 98115; 206-521-6001.

THE MOUNTAINEERS BOOKS, an active, nonprofit publishing program of the club, produces guidebooks, instructional texts, historical works, natural history guides, and works on environmental conservation. All books produced by The Mountaineers Books fulfill the club's mission.

Send or call for our catalog of more than 500 outdoor titles:

The Mountaineers Books
1001 SW Klickitat Way, Suite 201
Seattle, WA 98134
800-553-4453
mbooks@mountaineersbooks.org
www.mountaineersbooks.org

 The Mountaineers Books is proud to be a corporate sponsor of Leave No Trace, whose mission is to promote and inspire responsible outdoor recreation through education, research, and partnerships. The Leave No Trace program is focused specifically on human-powered (nonmotorized) recreation.

Leave No Trace strives to educate visitors about the nature of their recreational impacts, as well as offer techniques to prevent and minimize such impacts. Leave No Trace is best understood as an educational and ethical program, not as a set of rules and regulations.

For more information, visit www.lnt.org, or call 800-332-4100.

OTHER TITLES YOU MIGHT ENJOY FROM THE MOUNTAINEERS BOOKS

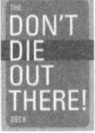

Don't Die Out There Deck
A compact, full deck of playing cards, with critical outdoor survival tips on each card

Backcountry Cooking Deck: 50 Recipes for Camp & Trail
Dorcas Miller
Delicious trail-ready recipes in a portable format (4x5$^1/_2$)

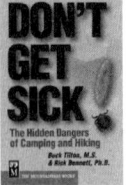

Don't Get Sick: The Hidden Dangers of Camping and Hiking
Buck Tilton & Rick Bennett
"[This] book will take up almost no space, but just might help you avoid big trouble, even death."—*Dayton News*

Don't Forget the Duct Tape: Tips & Tricks for Repairing & Maintaining Outdoor & Travel Gear, 2nd Edition *Kristin Hostetter*
"... a must-have for anyone whose outdoor gear gets loved to death on a regular basis."
—*The Flint Journal*

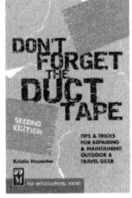

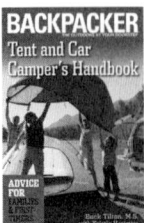

Tent and Car Camper's Handbook: Advice for Families & First-Timers
Buck Tilton, with Kristin Hostetter
"From the absolute basics to the details that can make a good experience great, these authors know their stuff and are eager to share it. Their love and respect for nature is both evident and contagious, and this book is a pleasure to read." —*Newsday*

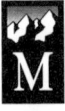

The Mountaineers Books has more than 500 outdoor recreation titles in print.
Receive a free catalog at
www.mountaineersbooks.org.